HOW TO GET RID OF AND CONTROL YOUR ECZEMA….

Your guide to controlling your Eczema, by understanding and acting upon the root causes of this skin condition.

Shelley Harding

Version 2
September 2012

CONTENTS

Terms of Use 4
About the author 5
How to control Eczema 6
Atopic eczema 7
Contact Eczema 12
Dyshidrotic Eczema 18
Hand Eczema 22
Seborrheic Eczema 26
Nummular eczema 29
Neuroeczema 31
Here's how to get started Controlling Eczema 34

TERMS OF USE

The content of this e-book is for information only and is not meant to replace consultation or advice from a qualified medical professional.

This e-book is intended for users who wish to research, learn, understand and collate information about controlling eczema. Nothing in this e-book should be considered personalized advice.

No part of this publication may be reproduced, stored in a retrieval system or transmitted in any form or by any means, electronic, mechanical, photocopying, recording, scanning or otherwise without the prior written permission of the author Shelley Rock.

Indemnity

You will indemnify and hold the e-book writer (hereinafter known as the "Indemnified Party") harmless from any breach of these Terms of Use by you, including any use of Content other than as expressly authorized in these Terms of Use. You agree that the Indemnified Party will have no liability in connection with any such breach or unauthorized use, and you agree to indemnify any and all resulting loss, damages, judgments, awards, costs, expenses, and attorney's fees of the Indemnified Party in connection therewith. You will also indemnify and hold the Indemnified Party harmless from and against any claims brought by third parties arising out of your use of the information in this e-book.

ABOUT THE AUTHOR

Shelley Harding is a health professional with many years experience helping people with eczema. On a personal note I have a special interest in eczema control since this is something my family has struggled with.

My eldest son and I were plagued by eczema and dry skin. For me the main areas of my body affected were my ears and the sides of my nose. When I had a flare up my ears and sides of my nose would look white and flake. When they got really dry they would crack and bleed. I bought every eczema product on the market as recommended by my doctor, but no matter how much I used the problem would not improve.

I would be especially embarrassed if I was at a function that went on for a while, because I knew that as time passed my ears and nose would look flaky again. And if I made the mistake of touching my itchy ears or my nose the flakes would deposit on my clothing making it look dirty and dusty.

Then one day it dawned on me that there must be something to the more neglected aspect of the underlying causes of eczema. I began to research this problem. During my research I discovered that people who found out the root causes of their eczema, and targeted these, had much better success getting rid of their eczema. I then began to pay closer attention to this, and when I started to target the root causes of my problem, my eczema improved considerably. When I ignored the root causes of my eczema, my eczema flared. Today my son and I live eczema free lives.

To learn more about eczema then click on the link below:

HOW TO CONTROL ECZEMA

How to control eczema is about helping people, who suffer from eczema to understand its causes, and drastically improve the quality of their lives.

Before you can control your eczema, you need to know the main triggers of your particular type of eczema.

If you follow these Simple tips, you will be able to find out the main triggers of your eczema condition and either improve the condition or eradicate it all together.

What is Eczema?

Eczema is a chronic skin condition which is triggered when your immune system has an over reaction to something in your environment, or when there is emotional stress. The skin may become dry, inflamed, scaly and itchy. In some persons there is a wet form of eczema, where there are watery boils that may weep and leave the skin soggy.

ATOPIC ECZEMA

Atopic eczema causes dry, itchy, irritated skin. Most people with atopic eczema develop it before age five. This skin condition tends to run in families. People who get atopic eczema usually have family members who have eczema, asthma, or hay fever.

Signs and Symptoms

- Usually the skin is dry and itchy, but this is not always so. In babies, patches develop on the scalp, face and cheeks. In older children and adults eczema patches tend to occur on the hands and feet. Other common sites for these patches are the bends of the elbows, backs of knees, ankles, wrists, face, neck, and upper chest. It should also be noted that while the above areas are the most common for eczema patches to occur on the skin, eczema can occur on any area of the body.

- The skin may become inflamed, cracked and weep, leading to the formation of a crust. The patches may be raised, scaly, dry and red. After the patches heal, a brown mark may be left. The skin may become thick with constant scratching. The scratching is usually in response to itching; and can lead to open sores and secondary infection.

A Baby with Atopic Eczema of the face

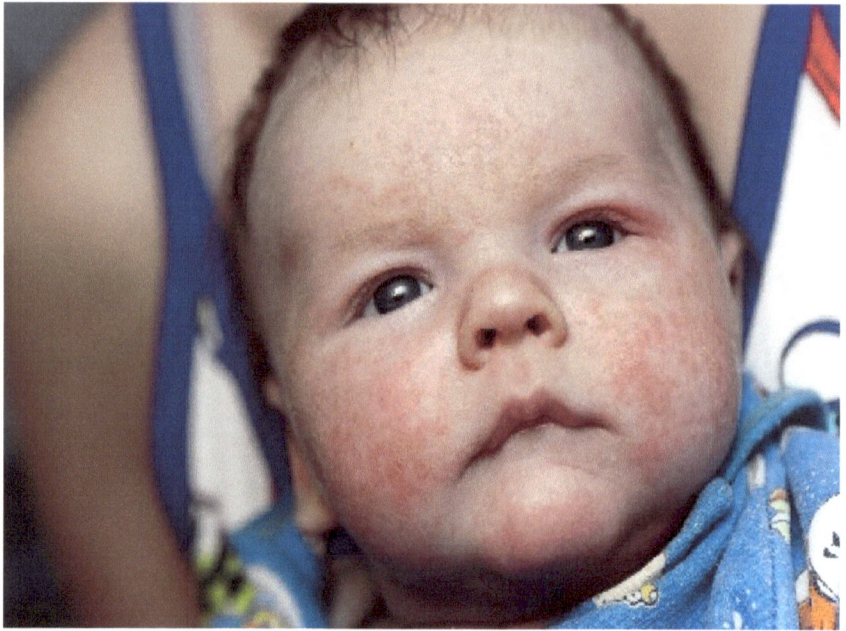

Causes

A large number of factors interact together to contribute to the development of atopic eczema. These include genetics, the home environment, damaged skin and a weak immune system.

Who is likely to get atopic eczema?

Family history. Those who have relatives with allergic type conditions such as atopic eczema, asthma, or hay fever; have the highest risk of developing atopic eczema. If one or both parents have the condition, then the child is more likely to develop it.

Living environment. It is well documented that those who live in urban polluted areas are more likely to get atopic eczema.

Age. More than 60 % of persons with atopic eczema develop it before the age of one year.

Sex. Females are slightly more likely to develop atopic eczema.

Social class. Atopic eczema is more common in those from higher social classes.

Areas of the Body Commonly Affected by Atopic Eczema

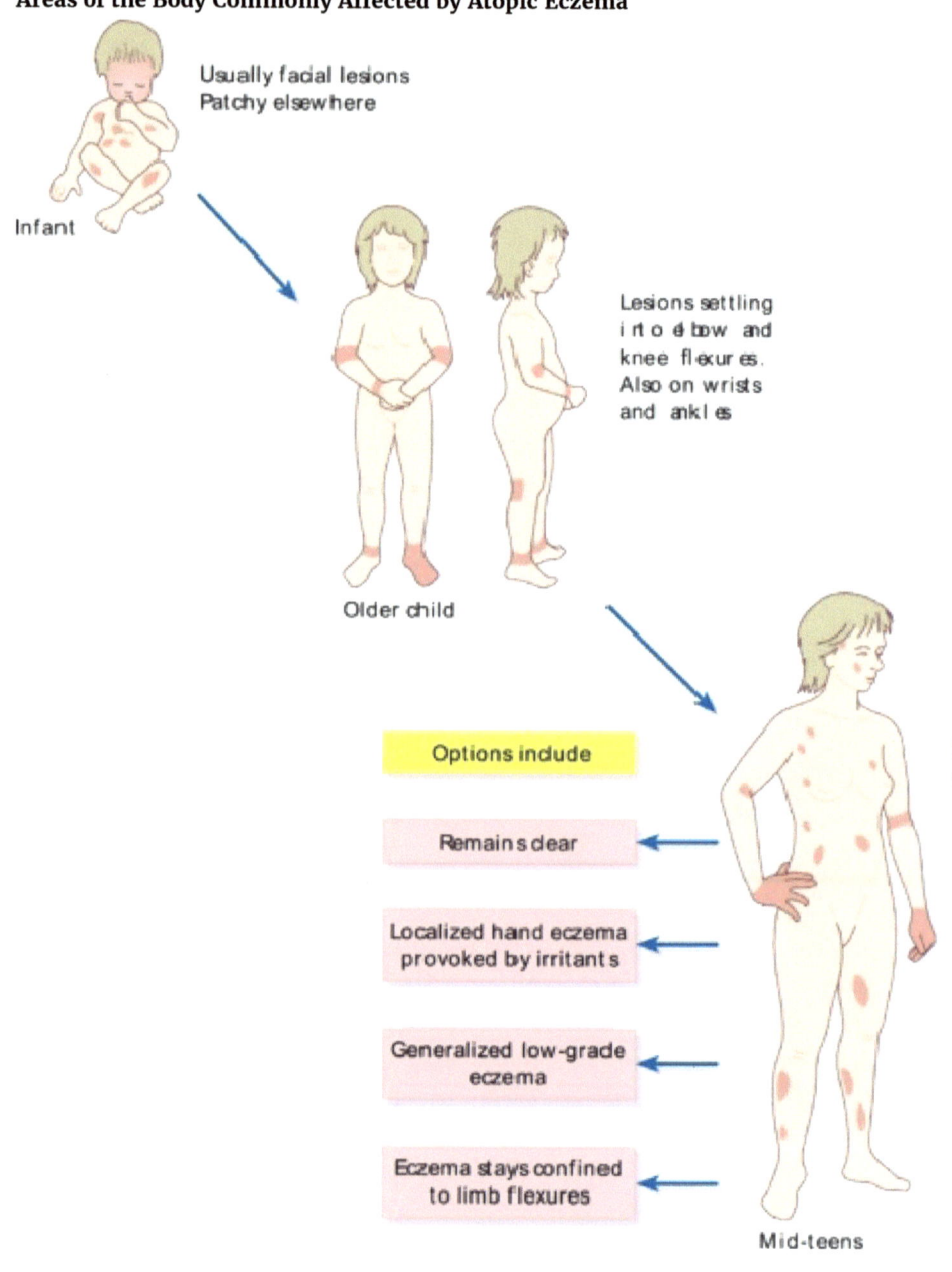

Living environment.
It is well documented that those who live in urban polluted areas are more likely to get atopic eczema.

Age. More than 60 % of persons with atopic eczema develop it before the age of one year.

Sex. Females are slightly more likely to develop atopic eczema.

Social class. Atopic eczema is more common in those from higher social classes.

CONTACT ECZEMA

Contact with everyday objects causes this very common type of eczema. When the contact leads to irritated skin, the eczema is called irritant contact eczema. If an allergic reaction develops on the skin after exposure, it is called allergic contact eczema.

Signs and Symptoms

Allergic contact eczema usually develops a few hours after the skin comes into contact with a substance to which the person is allergic. The following symptoms may occur:

- Itchy, swollen, and red skin or dry and bumpy skin

- Blisters may develop if the reaction is more severe

- Blisters may break, leaving crusts and scales

Skin may later flake and crack

- Long term exposure can lead to thick, red scaly skin, which may darken and become leathery over time.

Raised inflamed Eczema Patches on the feet

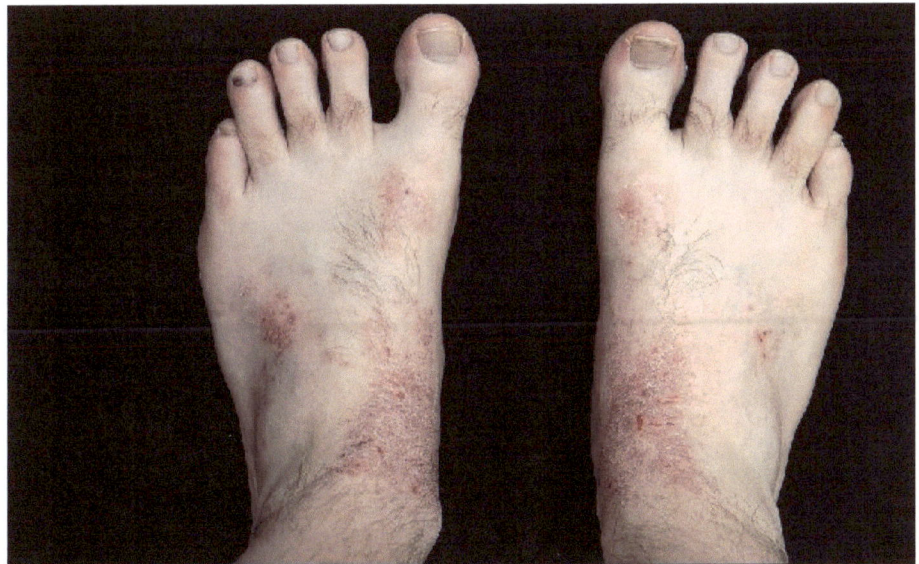

Irritant contact eczema occurs after frequent exposure to a mild irritant, such as dish washing liquid, and after brief exposure to a strong irritant, such as a strong acid.

Signs and symptoms of contact eczema caused by mild irritants include:
Patches of itchy, red, scaly, and swollen skin are characteristic of irritant contact eczema. The skin may burn or sting when it
comes into contact with the irritant. If exposure continues, the skin tends to crack, scale, and become excessively dry. Sores and blisters may develop and crusts and scales may form later.

Signs and symptoms of contact eczema caused by strong irritants:
Strong irritants may cause redness and swelling initially, and blisters and scales later.

Once irritant contact eczema develops exposure to mild substances, such as baby shampoo and even water, can irritate the skin and make the condition worse.

Causes

Allergic contact eczema. Many substances can cause allergic contact eczema. Common causes include:

- **Antibiotic ointment.** Ingredients in over-the-counter topical antibiotic ointments frequently cause an allergic skin reaction.

- **Clothing and shoes.** Materials and chemicals used in making clothing and shoes commonly cause allergic contact eczema.

- **Concrete.** Concrete causes contact eczema, especially on the hands. It may cause eczema on other parts of the body if the concrete dust gets inside the clothing.

- **Fragrances.** Fragrances are commonly found in toiletries ranging from make up to hair care products; and commonly cause allergies. It is also important not to assume that because

- the label on an item says unscented, it does not contain a fragrance. Some unscented products contain fragrances that are masked by additives which prevent the expression of the smell of the fragrance. It is therefore important to read the contents.

- **Metals.** Metals occur in everyday objects that we touch and in our food. Nickel, one of the most common metals that cause an allergic reaction, is found in jewellery and many foods. These include including nuts, and soy. Mercury, gold, cobalt, and also cause allergic contact eczema.

- **Plants.** Poison ivy and poison oak are frequent causes of allergic contact eczema.

    o **Rubber accelerators.** Rubber accelerators are chemicals used in the manufacturing of rubber. Almost all rubber products contain rubber accelerators. Below is a not exhaustive list of common products that contain rubber accelerators.

    o **Products Found in the Household**
o anti-slip carpet backing

- balloons
  - elastic bands
  - garden hoses and gloves
  - kitchen gloves
  - pillows and mattresses

- rubber gloves
- rubber handled sports equipment, e.g. golf club and racquet tennis racquet handles
- rubber handles (e.g. bicycles, car steering wheel)
- rubber kitchen utensils
- rubber swim caps and goggles

  - **Clothing and footwear**
- elastic in underwear and swimwear
- rubber boots
- sport shoes
- slippers
- rubber insoles of shoes
- elasticised waistbands
- brassiere cups

- **Cosmetics and healthcare products**
- rubber make-up sponges
- diaphragms
- rubber latex condoms
- thiuram is in the oral drug Antabuse (used to treat alcoholism)

  - **Products in the Workplace**
- commercial and agricultural fungicides and pesticides
- conveyor belts
- dental dams
- earphones
- elastic bandages

- electrical cords
- examination and surgical gloves

- gas masks
- lining for fuel tanks
- protective rubber aprons
- rubber hoses, seals and cables
- rubber mats
- rubber stoppers in medical syringes
- rubber tires and tubes
- safety goggles

- **Exposure to ultraviolet (UV) light**. Sunlight and other sources of ultra violet light may trigger the development of a rash. This is also known as photo allergy. This kind of contact eczema occurs when an every-day product such as skin lotion is applied to the skin, and then the skin is exposed to ultra violet light. Photo allergy may also occur during the time certain medications are being taken. Certain antibiotics such as ciprofloxacin, tetracycline and sulfamethoxazole, some malaria medications, and acne and cancer drugs may cause photosensitivity.

- **Perspiration**. In some persons perspiration triggers the rash of eczema. For example, some people will only develop a rash when nickel touches the skin, if they are perspiring at the same time.

Who is likely to get contact eczema?

- **Medical history**. Anyone can get contact eczema. However, as with most forms of eczema, having a history of allergic conditions increases the risk of getting contact eczema.

- **Age**. Younger persons tend to get contact eczema, because their immune system is more likely to overreact to allergens than older persons.

- **Repeat exposure**. Usually people develop contact eczema after repeated exposure to a particular thing. This is why it can be so difficult to identify the cause. A person may use something for years before they develop contact eczema as a result of its use. Mild irritants, such as detergent, require frequent exposure to cause irritant contact eczema.

- **Occupation**. People who work in certain occupations have a much higher risk of developing contact eczema. Health care workers, hairdressers, people who handle food, bartenders, janitors, and mechanics have an increased risk.

- **Environment**. Extreme heat and cold as well as very humid and very dry environments increase the risk.

Hands Damaged by Kerosene

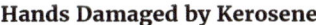

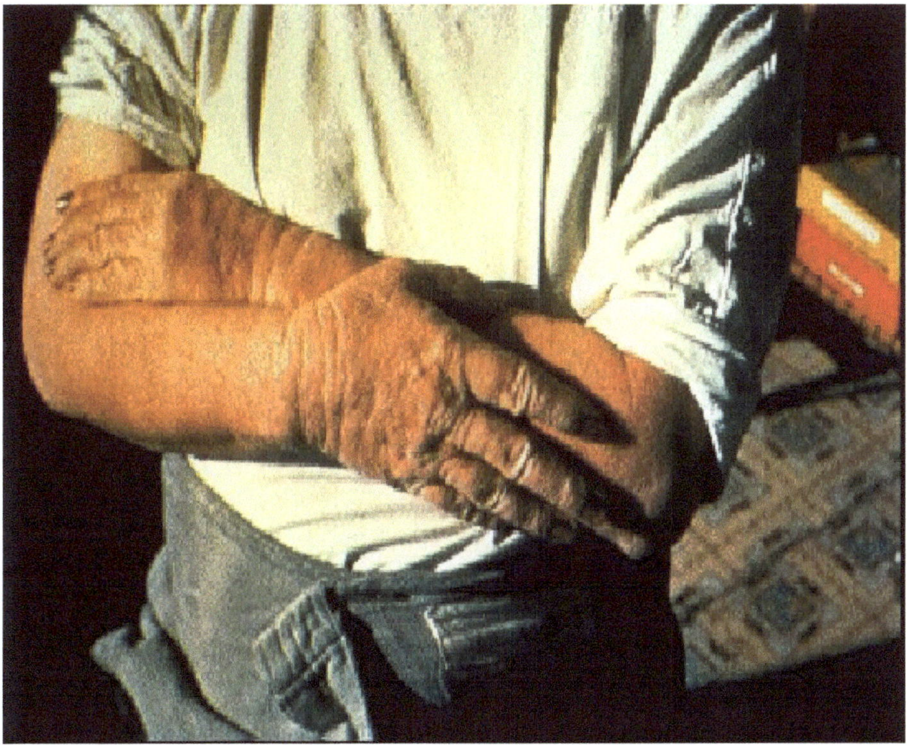

DYSHIDROTIC ECZEMA

- This occurs only on the palms of the hands, sides of the fingers, and soles of the feet. There is burning, an itching sensation and a blistering rash.

Signs and Symptoms

- Small, deep blisters can form on the palms, sides of the fingers, and/or soles of the feet
- Intense burning or itching
- Inflamed skin (reddish and hot to the touch)
- Cracking and peeling skin
- Skin may become infected, and may weep and form crusts
- The nails may become thick, ridged, pitted or discoloured.
- There may be extensive peeling and cracking.

Dyshidrotic Eczema of the Hands

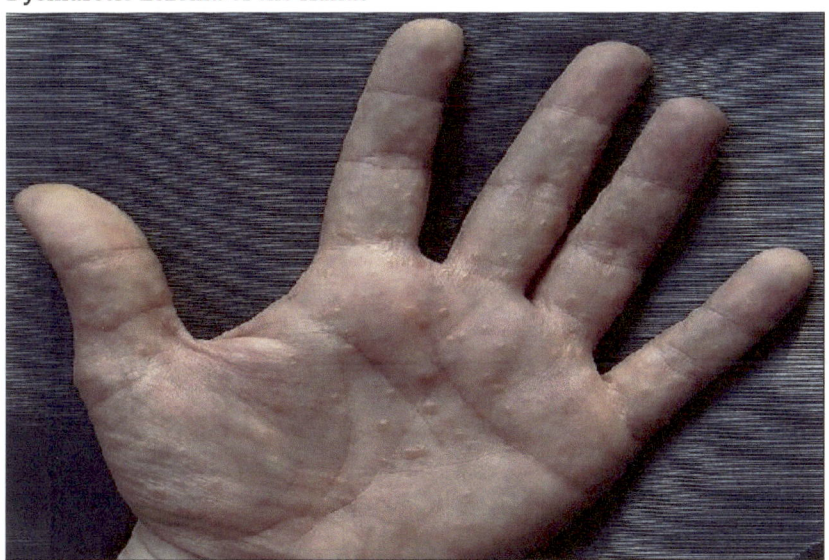

Extensive peeling and dryness with Eczema

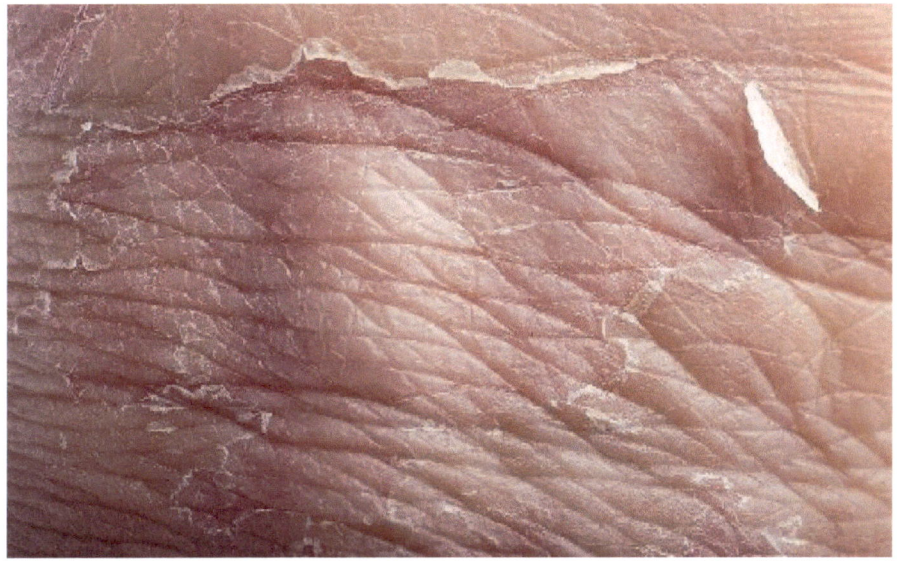

Who is likely to get dyshidrotic eczema?

- Mainly young adults, but may occur in older people. Rarely does it develop in children who have atopic eczema.

Causes

- **How Does Dyshidrotic Eczema Develop?**

No one knows for sure. However, it is thought that it is triggered by the immune response in people who have certain medical problems. Previously it was thought that the vesicles that develop on the skin were as a result of excessive sweating. It is now known that the fluid in the vesicles is sebum which collects between the outer layers of the skin. Sebum is an oily substance secreted by the sebaceous glands of the skin.

- **Stress.** Many people report a stressful episode before an outbreak of dyshidrotic eczema

- **Weather.** Dyshidrotic eczema is more common when the weather is hot and humid.

- **Pre-existing allergic conditions.** People with a history of allergies and allergic skin conditions are more likely to get dyshidrotic eczema.

- **Metal Allergy.** Dyshidrotic eczema is especially common in people with nickel allergy.

Dyshidrotic Eczema of the Feet

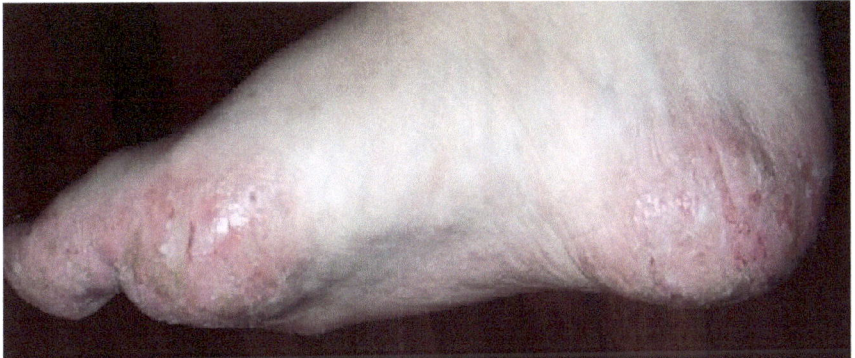

HAND ECZEMA

Signs and Symptoms

- Firstly, the hands become dry and chapped

- Later the skin become red, scaly and inflamed

- Itchy blisters or other lesions may form, skin may crack and weep

- Pus-filled lesions, crusting, and pain if skin becomes infected

- Can spread beyond the hands, particularly to the forearms and feet, if a skin infection develops or an allergic reaction is not treated

- Deformed nails when hand eczema persists for a long time.

Contact Eczema on the Hand

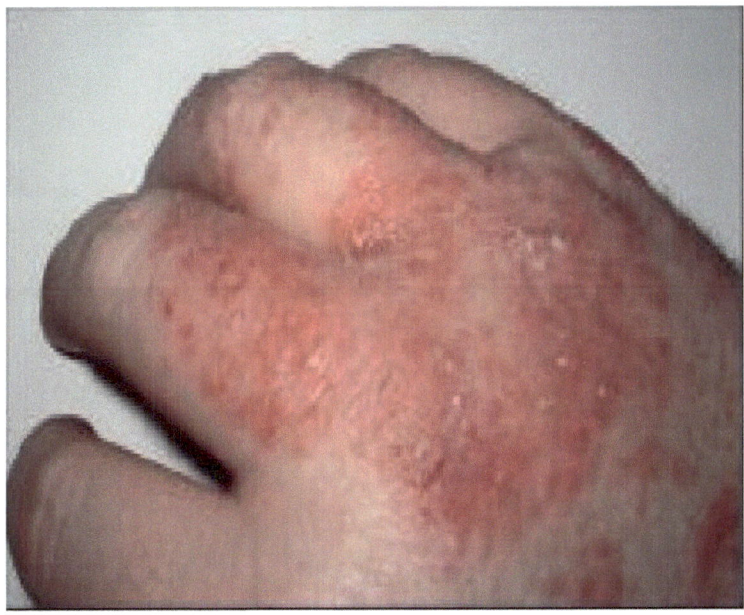

Who is likely to get hand eczema?

- Anyone can develop hand eczema

- Those working in occupations that involve constant hand washing or wearing of rubber gloves, e.g. dentists, nurses and hairdressers are more prone to develop hand eczema. It is also common in domestic cleaners and people whose occupation brings them into contact with harsh chemicals and metals.

- Having an allergy based condition such as asthma, hay fever, or atopic eczema, increases your chances of getting hand eczema.

Causes

Hand eczema usually does not have one clear-cut cause. It appears that many factors interact, including:

- **Genetics**. Hand eczema is more common in people with a family history of eczema

- **Irritation**. Repeated use or short intense exposure to every day items can cause hand eczema. Water is the most common irritant. Frequent use of water removes protective oils from the skin. This leaves the skin dry and less supple and more susceptible to eczema.

- **Allergy**. An allergic reaction occurs when the body's immune system overreacts to something that does not cause everyone's immune system to overreact. Common substances that can cause hand eczema include nickel, Balsam of Peru (added to

- fragrances, foods, and skin care products), rubber, and topical vitamin E

- **Gloves**. Some people are allergic to rubber and latex. Also constantly putting gloves on and off, can allow allergens to get into the gloves, causing irritation of the skin.

- **Stress**. Stress worsens all eczema. It is felt that stress affects the immune system negatively.

- **Environment**. Cold dry weather or hot humid weather increases the risk of developing hand eczema.

- **Excessive sweating**. When the hands sweat a lot, particularly when gloves are being worn.

Fingers severely damaged by Contact Eczema

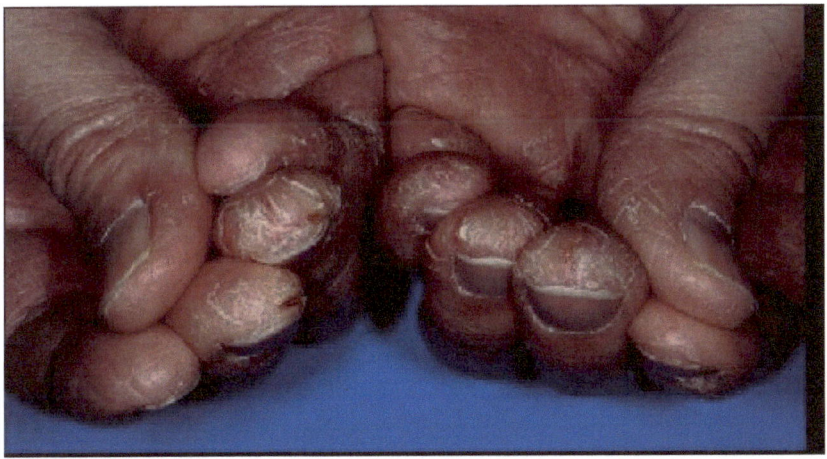

SEBORRHEIC ECZEMA

This is characterised by dry oily scales on the scalp. It commonly spreads to the forehead just beyond the hair line, the eye brows, around the nose and behind and inside the ears and the neck. It may also occur under the arms, under the breasts, the upper back, the navel, the groin and between the buttocks.

What Seborrheic eczema looks like?

- There is an oily, waxy appearance to the skin generally.

- The scale ranges in colour from white to yellowish brown depending on how oily the skin is.

- There may also be reddish raised areas of skin.

- The itching can be very severe. Constant scratching may lead to abrasions causing burning and secondary infection. This can lead to an itch scratch cycle where the more one scratches the more inflamed the skin becomes and the more one itches.

Causes of seborrheic eczema

It is felt that a number of things interact to cause seborrheic eczema. These are our genes, yeast on the skin, stress, the weather, and our generalhealth.

Severe Seborrheic Eczema on Scalp

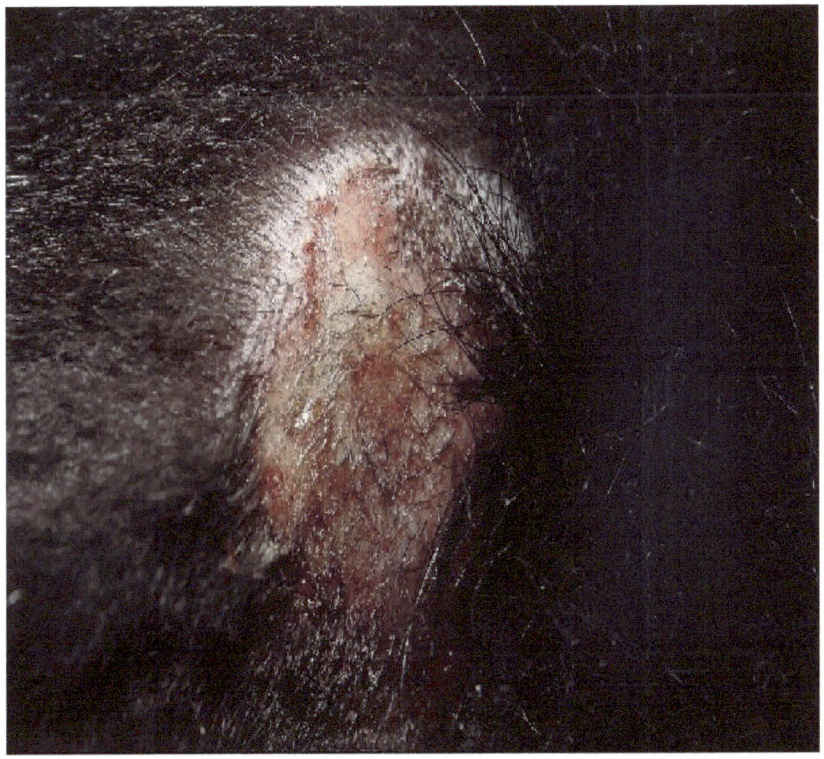

What makes us more likely to get Seborrheic Eczema?

- A family history of eczema
- Having oily skin or hair
- Stress
- Tiredness
- Cold, dry climate
- Being over weight
- Previous skin injury
- Products which dry the skin- e.g. medicated shampoos
- Having other skin conditions such as acne and psoriasis
- Taking certain medications.

Seborrheic Dermatitis of the Scalp

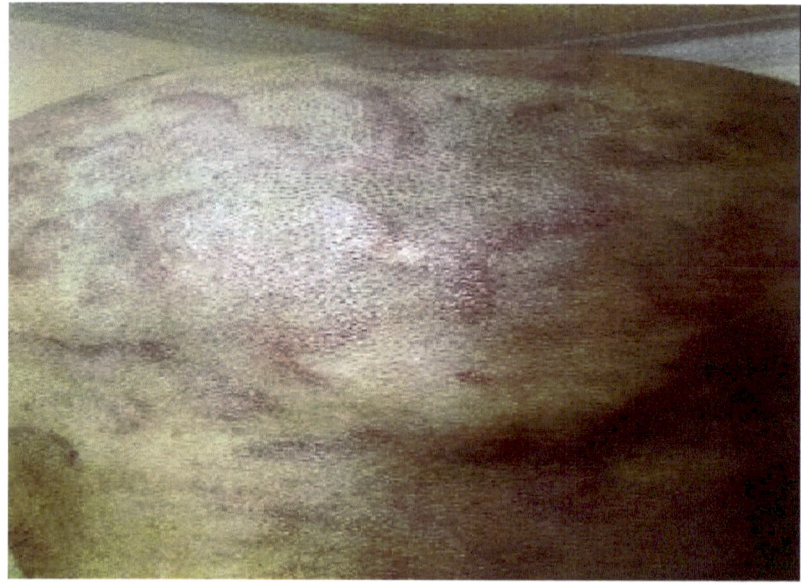

NUMMULAR ECZEMA

This usually presents as coin shaped or oval lesions on the skin.

They commonly occur after skin injuries, such as insect bites, burns and abrasions. The patches tend to develop on the hands, feet, legs and torso, but may occur any where on the skin.

What does Nummular Eczema look and feel like?

- One or many patches may appear.

    - They begin as small red spots and blisters that join together to become coin-shaped patches.
    - The patches range in size from about 1cm to 10 cm.
    - Recent patches may weep and become crusty. Later they become scaly
    - The patches always have a well defined edge which is sometimes raised, and when they clear in the centre they resemble ring worm.
    - The patches may be pink, red or brown.

- The patches may or may not itch.

- The skin between the patches is usually clear, but generally the skin is dry

- When the patches clear the skin may be lighter or darker than before.

- The patches may clear quickly, or take months to clear.

What contributes to the development of Nummular Eczema?

It is believed that heightened sensitivity to some substances contribute to the development of nummular eczema.

- **Mercury**. It is believed that in rare cases, exposure to mercury, which is a common component of dental fillings, can cause nummular eczema.

- **Rubber, nickel, formaldehyde, or neomycin**. If a person has an allergy to any of these, the skin will only clear when the substance is avoided.

Medical conditions. A history of very dry skin or eczema, especially atopic eczema or stasis eczema, increases the risk as does having poor blood flow and/or swelling in the legs.

- **Environment**. A cold dry environment.

- **Injury to the skin**. An insect bite, contact with chemicals, or an abrasion may trigger an outbreak.

- **Bacterial skin infection.** The rash may develop at the site of a bacterial infection.

- **Certain medications**. Isotretinoin, a prescription medication used to treat severe acne and interferon seem to trigger severe nummular eczema covering the entire body.

NEUROECZEMA

- Neuroeczema develops when nerve endings in the skin become irritated, triggering a severe itch-scratch-itch cycle. Common causes of nerve irritation include insect bites and emotional stress

What does the person with Neuroeczema experience?

- Intensely itchy skin that is usually itchiest when the person is resting or relaxing.
- Once the skin is scratched, a vicious itch-scratch-itch cycle develops. The more the skin is scratched, rubbed, or even touched, the more it itches. The itch can become so intense that it disrupts sleep.
- Neuroeczema develops on any area of the body the person can scratch or rub. It most commonly occurs on the lower legs, ankles, back and sides of the neck, wrists, forearms, and genitals.
- Constant itch causes anxiety in some persons.
- Often develops on skin previously affected by an outbreak of atopic eczema or contact eczema or psoriasis.

Scratching can cause:
- Small, well-defined, scaly, reddish plaques.
- Openings in the skin that cause burning pain and leave the person more susceptible to infection. Signs of infection include open sores, cracks in the skin, and honey-coloured crusts.
- Visible scratch marks.

- Over time, constant scratching causes the skin to thicken and darken, and lines in the skin to become more prominent. Thickening can cause a cutaneous horn (piling up of skin cells that resemble an animal's horn).
- Affected skin may turn pink, red, or reddish brown.

Who Gets Neuroeczema?

Neuroeczema develops more frequently in:
- People who have psoriasis, allergic contact eczema, or irritant contact eczema
- Individuals who have an atopic condition, such as atopic eczema, asthma, or hay fever
- Mainly women
- Mid-to-late adulthood, with most cases developing between 30 and 50 years of age

What contributes to the development of Neuroeczema?

Exposure to certain chemicals can trigger the development of neuroeczema. Research indicates that the following can irritate the nerves of susceptible people, triggering the intense itch-scratch-itch cycle of neuroeczema:
- Clothing worn tightly and made of synthetic fabric or wool
- Dry skin
- While uncommon, these may also trigger neuroeczema:
- Exhaust from traffic (long-term exposure)
- Exposure to skin irritants

- Heat
- Insect bite
- Period of intense stress or emotional trauma

- Poor blood flow
- Scar, especially a keloid-type scar

By now you should have a good idea of what type of eczema you have and the types of triggers associated with it. You are therefore well on your way to better control or elimination of your Eczema skin condition.

HERE'S HOW TO GET STARTED CONTROLLING ECZEMA

Step 1: Understand what triggers flare-ups of eczema

As you learned above, the triggers can be internal or external. Internal triggers are usually associated with things we ingest such as foods or inhale.

External triggers are things that come into contact with the skin, or environmental factors. These ranges from Physical and chemical irritants, extremes of temperature, humidity, perfumes, to different types of fabrics, and even detergents used to wash any clothing or linen that comes in contact with the skin. Stressful situations can also lead to flare ups of eczema in those so predisposed.

Avoid factors that cause eczema to worsen. Avoid exposure to dust and sand, wool and synthetic clothing materials, cigarette smoke and long hot baths or showers. If you live in areas with low humidity and rapid temperature changes use a humidifier in your home and layer your clothing so that you can easily adjust to the temperature in your surroundings.

Step 2: How to identify the triggers of

your eczema

The easiest way to do this is to keep a diary of all foods you ingest each day, places that you go which are associated with specific exposure, products you use on your skin, cleaning agent used in your environment and on the clothing you wear. It is important to be very detailed in itemizing your exposures. Do not forget to

record any stressful events or situations, as stress can trigger flare ups. You should then record the dates of any flare-ups of your eczema. After reviewing this over a period of time you will come to

notice what exposures preceded flare-ups of your eczema condition

Step 3: Remove the trigger identified above

If possible eliminate the trigger identified above from your environment. This can be difficult depending on the trigger.

If the trigger is a food, eliminating this food from your diet is easier than if it is the pollen from a particular plant that grows in the area where you live

Step 4: **Care of your skin**

Dry skin contributes to eczema and can cause it to become worse.

Cleanse the skin with gentle moisturizing cleansers and use warm, not hot water for your baths. Use natural moisturizers to keep the skin moist. Examples are body butters containing shea, almond, coconut, avocado and mango among others.

If the skin is broken or infected or you suffer from wet eczema you should consult your doctor.

Be gentle with your skin. Don't scratch it. Although eczema causes the skin to itch in the affected areas, scratching makes it worse. It can cause the skin to become thick, darker and to crack and bleed. Take precautions to try to minimize your scratching. Keep your fingernails cut short. If necessary, wear gloves at night to prevent scratching in your sleep.

Bathing and Moisturizing Guidelines

Bathing and moisturizing are essential for healthy skin. Bathing can hydrate skin, remove dirt and germs, and promote relaxation. It also can loosen crusts from inflamed skin. However, hot water, drying soaps, and rubbing to get skin clean or dry can aggravate eczema and cause a flare-up.

1. Use warm water for bathing and washing hands. You should use warm and not hot water to cleanse the skin. Hot water dries the skin. When the skin becomes dry, you are more prone to have a flare up of eczema.

2. Avoid excessive bathing. Bathing too frequently especially in hot water can dry the skin. A short warm shower or bath once a day, is important to hydrate the skin externally. When baths are avoided this contributes to the skin becoming dry.

3. Use mild, non-drying cleansers. Because eczema is a dry skin condition, it is important to use gentle cleaning agents, which do not strip the skin of its natural oils. Use natural mild cleansers that are free of chemicals, fragrances and additives.

Pay attention to the condition of your skin after using the cleanser.

If the skin does not feel smooth and moisturized, or becomes
irritated, change your cleanser. It is important to remember, that on an individual basis, every natural mild cleanser will not agree with your skin.

4. Avoid the use of ordinary soap. This is so important that it deserves to be mentioned on its own. Ordinary soap dries the skin by stripping it of its natural oils. Use gels or non-soap based cleansers to clean the skin; since these do not strip away natural oils.

5. Avoid the use of body sponges and washcloths. Body sponges and washcloths cause friction. This has two effects. It helps to strip away the skin's natural oils and irritates the skin.

6. Pat skin dry with a towel. Do not rub the skin dry. Rubbing skin dry with a towel removes important natural oils, and the moisture from the bath. Use your towel to pat the skin partially dry.

7. Apply moisturizer while the skin is damp. Applying moisturizer while the skin is damp locks in the moisture from the bath. In the winter, or when the air is dry, apply a heavy layer of moisturizer any areas of the skin that are exposed.

8. Select moisturizers with care. When selecting moisturizers, it is important to know a bit about them so that you can select the

ones that are best for you. It is important to know that moisturizers do not hydrate the skin, but helps to lock in the skin's own moisture. The more oil a moisturizer contains the better it protects against moisture loss. Moisturizers that come in ointment form contain the most oil. Ointments form a protective layer on the skin, and this makes them better moisturizers than creams and lotions. Ointments are especially good at preventing moisture loss when

the air is dry. Ointments should not be used on areas of the body that tend to get hot and sweaty. The next highest oil content is found in creams, followed by lotions. Water is the main ingredient in lotions, so lotions offer less protection against moisture loss than ointments and creams.

When selecting a moisturizer, be sure to keep in mind:

- That when the environmental air is dry, you need a moisturizer with high oil content. Body butters made from natural products are especially good when the environment is dry. Extra virgin cold presses varieties are especially good, because of the retention of their healing properties.

- When the air is moist, the skin can soak up moisture from the air. In this situation a lotion may be all that is needed.

- Use moisturizers that agree with your skin. You can be allergic to some of the contents of moisturizers. This is especially so

- with synthetic products that contains additives.

- Avoid moisturizers that contain perfumes, preservatives, and other chemicals that can irritate the skin.

Preventing Flare-Ups

Finding out what is causing your eczema and avoiding coming into contact with it is the most important step in controlling your eczema. There after following the steps below, can help you to avoid flare ups of your eczema.

1. Moisturize your skin. The main symptoms of skin prone to eczema are dryness and itching. Properly moisturizing the skin is one of the best ways at keeping eczema symptoms away.

The best way of locking in the skin's moisture is to apply your moisturizer immediately after your bath, to slightly damp skin.

It is also important to realise that you must also moisturize your skin internally. It is very important to drink adequate amounts of water each day. In fact, the water that you drink on a daily basis is the most important source of moisture for your skin.

2. Limit contact with skin irritants. The way we live now, means that we can come into contact with many different things during the course of a day. Find out what irritates your skin and limit contact with it. Avoid toiletries that contain things that dry the skin. The main offenders are products containing alcohol and soap.

3. Minimize sweating and keep cool. The itch/scratch cycle is usually triggered when you become hot and sweaty. Try to avoid situations that contribute to this. If you cannot, then have a cool
bath as soon as possible after the event and apply your moisturizer.

4. Keep an eye on temperature and humidity. Sudden rises in the temperature can cause you to become hot and sweaty, and
falls in the moisture of the air can cause your skin to become dry. Always be aware of the temperature and moisture content of the environment you are in, so that you can readily take steps to counteract any negative effects on your skin.

5. Take steps to avoid Scratching. Scratching makes the condition worse and may puncture skin allowing bacteria to enter and cause an infection. Gently applying a cold compress to the area that itches can reduce inflammation and lessen the desire to scratch.

6. Keep fingernails short. Short nails decrease the likelihood that scratching will damage the skin. Keep the nails short and wear cotton gloves at night to prevent any scratching from damaging the skin. Damaged skin is more prone to bacterial infection.

7. Dress in loose-fitting cotton clothes. Synthetic fabrics and wool can irritate the skin. Cotton clothing is soft and less likely to irritate the skin.

8. **Laundry tips.** Laundry detergents can trigger eczema flare-ups. Use hypoallergenic detergents where possible. Biological detergents tend to irritate the skin less. If hypoallergenic or non-bio detergents are unavailable, rinse clothing twice, to remove as much of the residue of the detergent as possible. Avoid fabric softeners, as most contain fragrances which can irritate the skin. Wash new clothing before wearing, to remove as much of the

excess dyes and chemicals used in making the material as possible.

9. **Watch out for stress.** Many people who suffer with eczema report that they get flare ups during stressful periods. It is important to remember that not only unpleasant experiences, like the loss of a job or loved one creates stress, but all life changing experiences creates a level of stress. To this end, things such as getting a promotion at work, moving into your dream house or getting married creates stress. It is important to recognise when
you are under stress, so that you can take steps to reduce your stress levels. This is something that you may want to get help with.

10. **Do not ignore medical advice.** Currently there are lots of natural treatments for eczema. There is also a lot of proof that these natural methods have helped many people get rid of their eczema. There are occasions when eczema is very severe, or the skin becomes infected with bacteria. It is very important to seek medical advice in these cases. Strong medications which are only available on prescription may be needed to treat severe cases of eczema. In addition if damaged eczema skin becomes infected,
antibiotics will be needed to clear up the infection. Infected skin left untreated can lead to very serious and sometimes life threatening illness.

Important food groups to make a part of your regular diet.

Before we look at the process, let us take a look at the types of foods that are important for a healthy immune system, and that will improve health overall. This is not new material, but is the brainchild of Professor Edmund Szekely. He classified foods into four categories depending on their qualities and what they contributed to one's health.

Biogenic: life renewing foods

The word biogenic refers to foods that are capable of generating a new living organism on their own. They mainly consist of different types of seeds. Examples of these are germinated cereal seeds, nuts and sprouted baby greens and legumes. These foods provide the proteins necessary to build strong body tissues.

Bioactive: Life sustaining foods

These foods are not capable of generating a new organism, but contain nutrients that can sustain life. Bioactive foods are natural unprocessed foods such as organic, natural vegetables and fruits.

It is felt that together, bioactive and biogenic foods synthesize substances that the body needs to function at its best. They contribute to the building of haemoglobin in the blood that serves to transport oxygen. They contribute other essential nutrients that promote cell respiration and biological resistance. They help to accelerate cell renewal and stimulate the natural self healing process. Bioactive and biogenic foods are more beneficial to the body when eaten raw.

Biostatic: Life slowing foods

Cooked foods and those that are not fresh (legumes must be cooked after sprouting first) are known as biostatic foods. These foods slow down the body's ability to regenerate and repair itself; and accelerate the aging process.

Biocidic: Life destroying foods

These are foods that have been refined and processed. They contain harmful substances such as chemicals, additives, and preservatives. We should only eat foods form the biogenic and bioactive groups.

The foods to avoid

- Eliminate any food from which vital nutrients have been removed. The list is long here, but these include foods made with white flour and white sugar.

- Do not use any food that the natural state has been altered. Processing destroys vital nutrients.

- Avoid foods that have been preserved, canned, frozen or ripened artificially. These processes cause depletion or complete destruction of vitamins, enzymes and plant hormones.

- Avoid foods that contain synthetic additives such as chemical preservatives, anti-oxidants, humectants, emulsifiers and colourings among others. Some of these substances are carcinogenic.

- Avoid artificial substitutes of natural foods.

- Avoid using foods that have been stored for a long time. Even biogenic and bioactive foods will loose their nutritive value after being stored for long periods of time.

The foods that should be a part of your regular diet

- Fresh raw fruits and vegetables

- Organic fruits and vegetables, whole grains, seeds, beans, nuts, yoghurt, fresh organic eggs, fresh organic milk.

- Avoid meat.

Your daily diet should consist of 25% biogenic foods, 50% bioactive foods and 25% biostatic foods. No biocidic foods should be consumed. Just following the above advice will greatly improve, not just your eczema, but also your general health.

What to buy at the Food Store

Now that you know what types of foods are good for you, and which are detrimental to your general health, the next task is to choose wisely when you shop for foods. Plan what you want for breakfast lunch and dinner. Make a list of the foods you want to get from each list with some recipes in mind and stick to that.

Get fresh foods, rather than those that have been treated or processed in a way that changes their natural state. For example, fresh coconut is packed with nutrients and vitamins, desiccated coconut, coconut that has been dried and preserved, has had its nutritional value destroyed. When shopping, buy the fresh coconut, rather than the desiccated one.

You want your diet to be balanced, so make sure you get a good blend of the major food groups. Remember that fresh ingredients, or ingredients that have not been treated in any way provide the best nutritional value. Try to buy organic as much as possible. Since these can be expensive, try planning your menu around what is seasonal. Avoid packaged foods like cereals, soups, frozen foods and powder mixes.

Examples of Foods that you can use in your Diet
Biogenic foods- (Proteins, carbohydrates, vitamins, minerals)
1. Nuts- hazel nuts, Brazil nuts, walnuts, almonds, pecan nuts, pistachios.
2. Sprouting seeds- bean sprouts, wheat, rye, radish, lentils, garlic
3. Raw cheeses- goat, cow
4. Fermented dairy products- organic yoghurt, cottage cheese.

Bioactive foods- (Antioxidants, vitamins, minerals, carbohydrates)
1. Raw fresh organic fruits- apples, oranges, bananas, strawberries, pineapples, blueberries, avocados, melons etc
2. Raw fresh organic vegetables- cucumbers, tomatoes, carrots, lettuce, spinach, cabbage, bell peppers, onions, garlic etc.
3. Dried fruits without preservatives- apricots, sultanas, raisins, pineapple, bananas, pears etc.

Biostatic foods- (carbohydrates, proteins, vitamins, minerals)
1. Organic brown rice
2. Organic potatoes
3. Organic Beans- Kidney beans, chickpeas, pinto, butterbeans etc
4. Organic whole grains- Millet, wheat, rye, spelt, cous cous etc

5. Organic cooking vegetables- Broccoli, kale, carrots, cabbage, onions etc

Seasonings and Dressings
1. Cold pressed organic oils- olive oil, coconut oil, flaxseed oil etc
2. Organic non-irradiated spices, organic mustard and Celtic salt for seasoning
3. Organic raw honey, organic jellies, pure maple syrup

The above list of foods is not exhaustive, but is designed to get you started. As much as possible buy what is seasonal in your local area, as this will cost you less. They will also be fresher and of greater nutritional value. Aim for organically produced products that have not been processed in a way that destroys their nutritional value.

Improve your Eczema by Eating Right

Over the years, much has been said about eczema and diet. There has also been the recognition that certain foods are immune system boosters. There has also been the recognition that some foods trigger bouts of eczema in some people. It follows, that the subject of eczema and food has been researched by people looking for relief from eczema.

This section takes you through a process that will help you to get rid of your eczema speedily. However, this is not for every one. You should not follow this process, if you are pregnant, have diabetes, conditions that require special dietary protocols, such as enzyme deficiencies; or suffer from liver or kidney disease. In the event that you may not be aware that you have any of the conditions mentioned above, you should have a medical check up first, before starting this process, even if you are healthy.

There are two parts to this process, first you get rid of the toxins in your body that contribute to flare-ups of eczema, and then you follow a 10 day diet designed to replenish the body, and solidify the benefits of the apple detoxification process. After this you should then follow a healthy diet as outlined above.

Some people may feel unwell during the detoxification process, and may want to skip this. Also you may have medical problems that will make it dangerous for you to try this process. If that is the case, skip the detoxification process, and just go right on to eating

a healthy diet as outlined above. Over time you will still see an improvement in your eczema. However, this will take a longer time that if you were able to use the detoxification process first.

The Detoxification process

There are many detoxification processes out there; however, one of the best is the apple detoxification method. The detoxification process allows you to rid your body of the harmful toxins and bacteria that have built up over the years. During the process, your body will eject toxins via your stool, urine and sweat. The detoxification process takes about 2-3 days. During this time you should not eat or drink anything other than water that has not been chemically treated.

During the 2-3 day period you should eat nothing except raw organic apples. Since you will only be surviving on apples you should eat lots of them, to supply you with the energy you need and to satisfy your hunger. If you do this you are less likely to feel unwell during this process. Remember, the reason you are doing this is to rid your body of toxins, **it is not a fast**.

The main reason why people may feel unwell during this process is that they are not getting enough energy to supply their needs. It is important to avoid this by eating lots of apples. Try to eat a variety of different apples to vary the taste, and make it more interesting. Apples are chosen because they contain a range of nutrients. Importantly they contain sugars to give you emery.

They also contain a wide range of vitamins and minerals, such as
vitamins A and C, magnesium, calcium, iodine, iron, and potassium.

Towards the end of the 2-3 day detoxification process, you may experience the following effects:
1. Headaches
2. lose bowels
3. mood swings

4. upset stomach

These effects are the sign that your body is working to flush out the harmful toxins. Because we are individuals every one may not experience these; and for some they will be more severe than for others.

The 10 day Cleanse and Replenish Diet

Immediately after the 2-3 day detoxification process, you need to go right on to the 10 day cleanse and replenish diet. What follows is a guideline to the types of things you should eat during this period, and the combinations of foods that you should avoid. You are therefore free to vary the specifics, as long as you stick to biogenic, bioactive and a minimum of biostatic foods. You will need a food processor and a juicer.

Here are the rules to follow for your 10 day diet

1. **Breakfast**- Breakfast should consist of organic fruits only; eat as much as you want. I.e., no other types of foods should be consumed with your fruits at breakfast.
2. Do not eat proteins and starches together, as they require two different types of enzymes to digest them. As a reminder, proteins are foods such as eggs, dairy, nuts and beans. Starches are foods such as brown rice, and potatoes.
3. Eat one large biogenic meal each day. Ensure that this meal contains sprouted seeds and grains. Remember biogenic foods are foods such as Nuts- hazel nuts, Brazil nuts, walnuts, almonds, pecan nuts, pistachios; sprouting seeds- bean sprouts, wheat, rye, radish, lentils, garlic.
4. Drink 2 glasses of carrot juice daily. This aids the skin healing process.

5. Do not eat any biocidic foods. These are foods such as white bread, sugar, coffee and all processed pre-packaged foods.

6. Eat limited amounts of biostatic foods. These include cooked vegetables, dairy products, fish and chicken.

After you have done this for 10 days, to continue to benefit it is a good idea to stick to the basic rules and to continue to avoid biocidic foods as much as possible.

Congratulations! You are on your way to taking control of your eczema condition

Disclaimer
The information in this e-book is meant for information only.
Persons suffering with eczema should always obtain the advice of a registered health care professional.

References:
MedicineNet Search
e-How.co.uk
Contact Allergens-DermnetNZ.org

Thank you for reading this e-book.

www.ingramcontent.com/pod-product-compliance
Lightning Source LLC
Chambersburg PA
CBHW041206180526
45172CB00006B/1208